10-minute diabetic diet cookbook after 50

Ultimate Guide To 2000+ Days Of Nutritious And Tasty Low-Carb, Low-Fat, Low-Suagr Recipes Suitable For Prediabetes, Type 2 Diabetes, With A 31-Day Meal Plan

Angelo Melvin

Table of Contents

COPYRIGHT © 2023

CHAPTER ONE

Introduction to Quick Diabetic Cooking After 50

Managing diabetes becomes increasingly crucial as individuals age, particularly for seniors over the age of 50. Among the myriad challenges they face, one significant concern is maintaining a balanced diet that not only manages blood sugar levels effectively but also fits into their lifestyle. Quick diabetic cooking emerges as a practical solution, offering seniors the ability to prepare nutritious meals in a time-efficient manner. This comprehensive guide explores the importance of quick meals for seniors managing diabetes, elucidates the benefits of time-efficient cooking for older adults, and provides essential tips for fast and healthy cooking after 50.

Importance of Quick Meals for Seniors Managing Diabetes

For seniors managing diabetes, the significance of quick meals cannot be overstated. As age advances, various factors such as mobility issues, fatigue, and cognitive decline can make meal preparation challenging. Additionally, the need for adherence to dietary restrictions to control blood sugar levels further complicates the process. Quick meals offer several advantages in addressing these challenges:

- Convenience: Quick meals require minimal time and effort to prepare, making them ideal for seniors with limited mobility or energy. With simple recipes and readily available ingredients, they can whip up a nutritious meal without exerting themselves excessively.

- Blood Sugar Management: Consistency in meal timing and portion control are essential for managing diabetes. Quick meals enable seniors to maintain regular eating schedules and adhere to portion sizes, thus helping stabilize blood sugar levels throughout the day.

- Variety: Quick cooking does not equate to bland or monotonous meals. Seniors can experiment with a wide range of ingredients and recipes, ensuring they enjoy diverse flavors and nutrients without compromising on convenience.

- Cost-Effectiveness: Eating out frequently or relying on pre-packaged meals can strain a senior's budget. Quick meals prepared at home are more economical, allowing seniors to save money while still enjoying delicious and healthy food.

- Independence: Being able to prepare quick meals empowers seniors to maintain their independence and autonomy in managing their health. Instead of relying on others for meal preparation, they can take charge of their diet and make choices that align with their preferences and nutritional needs.

In essence, quick meals play a vital role in simplifying the dietary management of diabetes for seniors, offering convenience, nutritional benefits, and the ability to maintain independence in meal preparation.

Benefits of Time-Efficient Cooking for Older Adults

Time-efficient cooking holds numerous benefits for older adults, particularly those over the age of 50 who are managing diabetes. These benefits extend beyond mere convenience and encompass various aspects that contribute to overall well-being:

- Healthier Choices: When pressed for time, individuals may resort to unhealthy convenience foods high in refined sugars and unhealthy fats. Time-efficient cooking encourages the use of fresh, wholesome ingredients, enabling seniors to make healthier food choices that support their diabetes management goals.

- Stress Reduction: Long, elaborate meal preparation can be stressful, especially for seniors with limited energy or mobility. Quick cooking techniques such as stir-frying, steaming, or using a pressure cooker help reduce cooking time and alleviate stress associated with meal preparation.

- Enhanced Nutrition: Quick cooking methods such as steaming and stir-frying retain more nutrients in foods compared to prolonged cooking methods like boiling. By minimizing cooking time, older adults can preserve the nutritional integrity of ingredients, ensuring they derive maximum health benefits from their meals.

- Time Savings: Time-efficient cooking allows seniors to free up valuable time for other activities they enjoy, such as socializing, exercising, or pursuing hobbies. By streamlining meal preparation, they can strike a balance between managing their diabetes and maintaining an active lifestyle.

- Improved Compliance: Complex recipes with long preparation times may discourage seniors from adhering to their dietary plans. Time-efficient cooking simplifies the cooking process, making it easier for seniors to comply with their diabetes management regimen consistently.

In summary, time-efficient cooking offers a multitude of benefits for older adults managing diabetes, including healthier food choices, reduced stress, enhanced nutrition, time savings, and improved compliance with dietary guidelines.

Essential Tips for Fast and Healthy Cooking After 50

To maximize the benefits of quick cooking for seniors managing diabetes, it's essential to adopt strategies that prioritize both speed and health. The following tips offer practical guidance for fast and healthy cooking after the age of 50:

- Meal Planning: Plan meals in advance to streamline the cooking process and ensure you have all the necessary ingredients on hand. Consider batch cooking or preparing components of meals in advance to save time during busy weekdays.

- Focus on Nutrient Density: Opt for nutrient-dense ingredients such as leafy greens, lean proteins, whole grains, and healthy fats. These foods provide essential nutrients while helping to regulate blood sugar levels and promote overall health.

- Embrace Simple Recipes: Choose recipes that require minimal ingredients and preparation steps. Look for quick and easy dishes that can be prepared in 30 minutes or less, utilizing cooking techniques like stir-frying, grilling, or oven-roasting for maximum efficiency.

- Utilize Time-Saving Kitchen Gadgets: Invest in kitchen gadgets such as pressure cookers, slow cookers, and food processors to expedite meal preparation. These appliances can significantly reduce cooking time while allowing you to create flavorful and nutritious meals with ease.

- Incorporate Frozen and Pre-Cut Ingredients: Frozen fruits and vegetables are convenient options that retain their nutritional value and require minimal preparation. Similarly, pre-cut vegetables and pre-cooked grains or proteins can expedite meal assembly without sacrificing quality or freshness.

- Opt for One-Pot Meals: Simplify cleanup and save time by preparing one-pot meals such as soups, stews, or casseroles. These hearty dishes can be packed with nutritious ingredients and customized to suit your taste preferences while minimizing cooking time and dishwashing chores.

- Experiment with Flavorful Seasonings: Enhance the taste of quick meals by experimenting with herbs, spices, and flavorful condiments. Fresh herbs, citrus zest, garlic, ginger, and low-sodium sauces can add depth and complexity to dishes without additional cooking time.

- Stay Hydrated: Drinking an adequate amount of water is essential for overall health, especially for seniors managing diabetes. Stay hydrated throughout the day to support digestion, metabolism, and blood sugar regulation, which can indirectly contribute to energy levels and well-being.

By incorporating these essential tips into your cooking routine, you can enjoy fast and healthy meals that support your diabetes management goals while catering to the unique needs and preferences of older adults.

CHAPTER TWO

Efficient Kitchen Setup for Quick Cooking

Creating an efficient kitchen setup is paramount for seniors aiming to prepare quick and healthy meals, especially when managing diabetes. A well-equipped and organized kitchen can streamline the cooking process, enhance safety, and promote independence. This section delves into essential kitchen tools and gadgets for seniors, strategies for organizing the kitchen for efficiency and safety, and tips for stocking the pantry with quick and healthy ingredients.

Essential Kitchen Tools and Gadgets for Seniors

Equipping the kitchen with essential tools and gadgets can significantly facilitate quick cooking for seniors. Here are some indispensable items tailored to meet the needs of older adults:

- Ergonomic Utensils: Opt for lightweight and ergonomic utensils with non-slip handles to facilitate comfortable grip and ease of use. Adaptive utensils with larger grips or angled handles can help alleviate strain on arthritic hands and promote independence in meal preparation.

- Electric Appliances: Invest in electric appliances that simplify cooking tasks, such as electric kettles, toaster ovens, and countertop grills. These appliances are user-friendly and require minimal manual effort, making them ideal for seniors seeking convenience and efficiency.

- Sharp Knives: Sharp knives are essential for efficient and safe meal preparation. Choose knives with ergonomic handles and blade guards to minimize the risk of accidents. Regularly sharpen knives to maintain their effectiveness and ensure smooth cutting.

- Microwave Oven: A microwave oven is a versatile appliance that enables seniors to quickly heat, defrost, or cook a variety of foods. Opt for a model with user-friendly controls and appropriate safety features, such as child lock and automatic shut-off.

- Food Processor or Blender: A food processor or blender can streamline tasks such as chopping vegetables, pureeing sauces, or blending smoothies. Choose a model with accessible controls and easy-to-clean components for added convenience.

- Non-Stick Cookware: Non-stick cookware reduces the need for excess oil or fat during cooking and facilitates easy cleanup. Select pots and pans with sturdy handles and heat-resistant coatings to ensure durability and safety.

- Digital Kitchen Scale: A digital kitchen scale is indispensable for precise ingredient measurement, particularly when following recipes or adhering to dietary guidelines. Look for a scale with large, easy-to-read display and intuitive controls for user-friendly operation.

- Can Opener: A reliable can opener is essential for seniors who frequently use canned ingredients in their cooking. Choose a manual or electric can opener with ergonomic handles and smooth cutting action for effortless operation.

By outfitting the kitchen with these essential tools and gadgets, seniors can enhance efficiency, safety, and enjoyment in their cooking endeavors, paving the way for quick and hassle-free meal preparation.

Organizing Your Kitchen for Efficiency and Safety

Efficient organization of the kitchen is crucial for optimizing workflow, minimizing clutter, and ensuring safety, especially for seniors. Follow these tips to organize your kitchen effectively:

- Declutter Countertops: Clear clutter from countertops to create ample workspace for meal preparation. Store frequently used items within easy reach and reserve countertop space for essential appliances and tools.

- Arrange Cabinets and Drawers: Arrange cabinets and drawers strategically to facilitate easy access to cooking essentials. Group similar items together and use drawer organizers or dividers to keep utensils and gadgets neatly organized.

- Prioritize Accessibility: Store frequently used items at eye level or within arm's reach to minimize bending or stretching. Reserve lower cabinets for lightweight or seldom-used items, and use step stools or reach extenders for accessing high shelves safely.

- Ensure Adequate Lighting: Adequate lighting is essential for visibility and safety in the kitchen, particularly for seniors with vision impairments. Install bright, energy-efficient lighting fixtures above work areas and task lighting under cabinets for optimal illumination.

- Implement Safety Measures: Minimize hazards in the kitchen by implementing safety measures such as securing loose rugs or mats, installing grab bars near cooking surfaces, and using non-slip mats under appliances and cutting boards.

- Label Ingredients and Containers: Label ingredients and containers clearly to facilitate easy identification and prevent confusion during meal preparation. Use large, high-contrast labels with clear text for optimal readability, especially for seniors with visual impairments.

By organizing the kitchen with efficiency and safety in mind, seniors can streamline meal preparation, reduce stress, and enhance their overall cooking experience, allowing them to focus on enjoying delicious and nutritious meals.

Stocking Your Pantry with Quick and Healthy Ingredients

A well-stocked pantry is essential for quick and convenient meal preparation, providing seniors with access to a variety of ingredients for nutritious and flavorful dishes. Here are some essential pantry staples for quick cooking:

- Whole Grains: Stock up on whole grains such as brown rice, quinoa, oats, and whole wheat pasta for a nutritious foundation to meals. These grains are rich in fiber and complex carbohydrates, which help stabilize blood sugar levels and promote satiety.

- Canned Beans and Legumes: Canned beans and legumes, such as chickpeas, black beans, and lentils, are convenient sources of protein, fiber, and essential nutrients. Rinse canned beans before use to reduce sodium content and enhance digestibility.

- Canned Tomatoes: Canned tomatoes are versatile pantry staples that can be used to create flavorful sauces, soups, and stews. Opt for low-sodium varieties and diced, crushed, or pureed tomatoes for added convenience.

- Healthy Oils: Choose heart-healthy oils such as olive oil, avocado oil, or coconut oil for cooking and salad dressings. These oils provide essential fatty acids and antioxidants while adding flavor and richness to dishes.

- Herbs and Spices: Stock a variety of herbs, spices, and seasoning blends to add depth and complexity to your meals without extra calories or sodium. Experiment with different flavor profiles to enhance the taste of your dishes.

- Nut Butter: Nut butter, such as almond butter or peanut butter, is a nutritious spread that can be used in sauces, smoothies, or as a topping for toast or fruit. Look for natural nut butter without added sugars or hydrogenated oils.

- Low-Sodium Broth or Stock: Keep low-sodium broth or stock on hand for soups, stews, and sauces. Choose vegetable, chicken, or beef broth depending on your preferences and dietary restrictions.

- Frozen Fruits and Vegetables: Frozen fruits and vegetables are convenient alternatives to fresh produce and retain their nutritional value. Stock up on a variety of frozen options for quick and easy additions to smoothies, stir-fries, and casseroles.

By stocking your pantry with these quick and healthy ingredients, you can simplify meal preparation, ensure access to nutritious foods, and create delicious meals with minimal effort. Experiment with different combinations and recipes to discover new flavors and culinary delights while supporting your diabetes management goals.

CHAPTER THREE

Speedy Breakfasts for Busy Mornings

Mornings can be hectic, especially for seniors managing diabetes who need a nutritious start to their day. Quick and convenient breakfast options are essential for maintaining energy levels and stabilizing blood sugar while navigating busy schedules. This section explores three speedy breakfast ideas tailored to busy mornings: quick and nutritious oatmeal variations, high-protein breakfast smoothies, and microwave egg muffins and breakfast wraps.

Quick and Nutritious Oatmeal Variations

Oatmeal is a versatile and nutritious breakfast option that can be customized to suit individual tastes and dietary preferences. Here are three quick and nutritious oatmeal variations to try:

- Overnight Oats: Prepare overnight oats the night before by combining rolled oats with your choice of milk (dairy or plant-based), yogurt, and toppings such as fresh fruit, nuts, seeds, or spices. Allow the mixture to soak in the refrigerator overnight, and enjoy a ready-to-eat breakfast in the morning. Experiment with different flavor combinations, such as cinnamon and apple or peanut butter and banana, to keep things interesting.

- Microwave Oatmeal: For a speedy breakfast option, microwave oatmeal is a convenient choice. Simply combine rolled oats, water or milk, and a pinch of salt in a microwave-safe bowl, and microwave on high for 2-3 minutes, stirring halfway through. Top with your favorite toppings, such as berries, sliced almonds, or a drizzle of honey, for added flavor and nutrition.

- Instant Pot Oatmeal: Utilize a pressure cooker like the Instant Pot to prepare oatmeal quickly and effortlessly. Combine oats, water or milk, and any desired flavorings or toppings in the Instant Pot, and cook on high pressure for 3-5 minutes, depending on the desired consistency. Allow the pressure to release naturally for a few minutes before opening the lid. Serve hot with a sprinkle of cinnamon or a dollop of yogurt for extra creaminess.

By incorporating these quick and nutritious oatmeal variations into your morning routine, you can enjoy a satisfying and wholesome breakfast without sacrificing precious time or compromising on taste.

High-Protein Breakfast Smoothies

Breakfast smoothies are a convenient and portable option for busy mornings, providing a quick and easy way to fuel your body with essential nutrients. Here are three high-protein breakfast smoothie recipes to try:

- Berry Blast Smoothie: Blend frozen mixed berries, spinach or kale, Greek yogurt, almond milk, and a scoop of protein powder until smooth and creamy. Add a tablespoon of chia seeds or flaxseeds for an extra boost of fiber and omega-3 fatty acids. Serve chilled in a tall glass or portable tumbler for a refreshing start to your day.

- Peanut Butter Banana Smoothie: Combine ripe bananas, creamy peanut butter, Greek yogurt, milk (dairy or plant-based), and a handful of ice cubes in a blender. Blend until smooth and frothy, adjusting the consistency with additional milk if necessary. For added sweetness, drizzle in a bit of honey or maple syrup. Garnish with a sprinkle of cocoa powder or chopped peanuts for an indulgent touch.

- Green Power Smoothie: Blend spinach or kale, frozen mango chunks, avocado, plain Greek yogurt, coconut water, and a squeeze of fresh lime juice until smooth and creamy. Add a handful of fresh mint leaves or a knob of ginger for extra freshness and flavor. Serve immediately in a chilled glass or mason jar for a revitalizing morning pick-me-up.

These high-protein breakfast smoothies are not only quick and easy to prepare but also packed with essential nutrients to keep you energized and satisfied throughout the morning.

Microwave Egg Muffins and Breakfast Wraps

Microwave egg muffins and breakfast wraps offer a protein-rich and portable breakfast option for busy mornings. Here's how to make them:

- Microwave Egg Muffins: Whisk together eggs, diced vegetables (such as bell peppers, spinach, onions, or mushrooms), and shredded cheese in a microwave-safe mug or ramekin. Microwave on high for 1-2 minutes, or until the eggs are set and cooked through. Serve hot with a side of whole grain toast or fresh fruit for a balanced meal.

- Breakfast Wraps: Fill whole grain tortillas or wraps with scrambled eggs, cooked turkey bacon or sausage, diced tomatoes, avocado slices, and a sprinkle of cheese. Roll up the wraps tightly and microwave for 30-60 seconds, or until heated through. Serve with salsa or Greek yogurt for dipping, if desired.

These microwave egg muffins and breakfast wraps are quick to prepare and can be customized with your favorite ingredients, making them an ideal choice for busy mornings when time is limited.

Incorporate these speedy breakfast ideas into your morning routine to start your day off right with a nutritious and satisfying meal that supports your diabetes management goals. Experiment with different variations and flavors to keep things exciting and enjoyable.

CHAPTER FOUR

Rapid Lunch Ideas for Midday Meals

Lunchtime can be a busy period, especially for seniors managing diabetes who require nutritious meals to sustain energy levels throughout the day. Quick and convenient lunch options are essential for maintaining blood sugar stability and supporting overall health. This section explores three rapid lunch ideas tailored to midday meals: simple salad and wrap recipes for seniors, protein-packed lunches for sustained energy, and easy soups and stews ready in minutes.

Simple Salad and Wrap Recipes for Seniors

Salads and wraps offer a versatile and refreshing option for quick lunches, providing a balanced combination of vegetables, protein, and healthy fats. Here are three simple salad and wrap recipes for seniors to enjoy:

- Classic Chicken Caesar Salad: Toss together chopped romaine lettuce, grilled chicken breast strips, cherry tomatoes, and shredded Parmesan cheese in a large bowl. Drizzle with Caesar dressing and toss until evenly coated. Serve with whole grain croutons on the side for added crunch.

- Veggie Hummus Wrap: Spread a whole grain tortilla or wrap with a generous layer of hummus, then layer with sliced cucumbers, bell peppers, carrots, avocado slices, and mixed greens. Roll up tightly and slice into bite-sized pinwheels for a portable and nutritious lunch option.

- Tuna Salad Lettuce Wraps: Mix together canned tuna, diced celery, red onion, mayonnaise, Dijon mustard, and a squeeze of lemon juice in a bowl. Spoon the tuna salad mixture onto large lettuce leaves, such as butter or romaine lettuce, and roll up to create lettuce wraps. Serve with a side of carrot sticks or cherry tomatoes for a satisfying and low-carb lunch.

These simple salad and wrap recipes are quick to prepare and can be customized with your favorite ingredients, making them an ideal choice for a rapid midday meal.

Protein-Packed Lunches for Sustained Energy

Protein-packed lunches provide sustained energy and help stabilize blood sugar levels, making them an excellent choice for seniors managing diabetes. Here are three ideas for protein-packed lunches:

- Quinoa Salad with Chickpeas and Feta: Combine cooked quinoa, canned chickpeas, diced cucumber, cherry tomatoes, red onion, and crumbled feta cheese in a large bowl. Drizzle with olive oil and lemon juice, then season with salt, pepper, and dried herbs such as oregano or thyme. Toss until well combined and serve chilled for a refreshing and satisfying lunch option.

- Turkey and Avocado Wrap: Spread a whole grain tortilla or wrap with mashed avocado, then layer with sliced turkey breast, baby spinach leaves, shredded cheese, and thinly sliced red bell pepper. Roll up tightly and slice into pinwheels for a protein-rich lunch that's perfect for on-the-go.

- Lentil Soup with Spinach and Sausage: Prepare a hearty lentil soup by simmering cooked lentils with diced Italian sausage, chopped spinach, carrots, celery, onion, garlic, and vegetable broth in a pot. Season with herbs and spices such as thyme, bay leaves, and smoked paprika for added flavor. Serve hot with a slice of whole grain bread or a side salad for a satisfying and nutritious lunch.

These protein-packed lunch ideas are not only delicious but also provide essential nutrients to support overall health and well-being, making them ideal for seniors managing diabetes.

Easy Soups and Stews Ready in Minutes

Soups and stews are comforting and nourishing lunch options that can be prepared quickly and easily. Here are three easy soup and stew recipes ready in minutes:

- Chicken and Vegetable Soup: Simmer diced cooked chicken breast, mixed vegetables, such as carrots, celery, and green beans, diced tomatoes, chicken broth, and cooked pasta or rice in a pot until heated through. Season with salt, pepper, and herbs such as parsley or thyme for a comforting and satisfying lunch option.

- Beef and Bean Chili: Brown ground beef or turkey in a pot, then add diced onion, bell pepper, garlic, canned kidney beans, diced tomatoes, tomato sauce, chili powder, cumin, and paprika. Simmer for 20-30 minutes until flavors meld and chili thickens. Serve hot with a dollop of Greek yogurt or shredded cheese for added creaminess.

- Vegetable Lentil Stew: Combine cooked lentils, diced potatoes, carrots, celery, onion, garlic, diced tomatoes, vegetable broth, and a bay leaf in a pot. Simmer until vegetables are tender and flavors develop, then season with salt, pepper, and herbs such as thyme or rosemary. Serve hot with a slice of crusty whole grain bread for a hearty and nutritious lunch.

These easy soup and stew recipes are perfect for busy days when you need a satisfying and wholesome meal in a hurry. Experiment with different ingredients and flavor combinations to suit your taste preferences and dietary needs.

Incorporate these rapid lunch ideas into your midday routine to enjoy delicious and nutritious meals that support your diabetes management goals. With a little planning and creativity, you can savor a variety of quick and convenient lunch options that keep you feeling satisfied and energized throughout the day.

CHAPTER FIVE

Fast and Flavorful Dinners After 50

As the day winds down, seniors managing diabetes still require nutritious and delicious dinners that are quick to prepare. Fast and flavorful dinner options are essential for maintaining a healthy diet while accommodating busy schedules. This section explores three types of dinners tailored to seniors after 50: one-pot meals for effortless cleanup, quick stir-fries and skillet dinners, and Instant Pot and slow cooker recipes for easy dinners.

One-Pot Meals for Effortless Cleanup

One-pot meals are a convenient and efficient dinner option, requiring minimal cleanup while still delivering delicious and nutritious meals. Here are three one-pot meal ideas for seniors:

- Chicken and Vegetable Quinoa: In a large pot or skillet, combine diced chicken breast, mixed vegetables (such as bell peppers, zucchini, and carrots), quinoa, chicken broth, and seasonings (such as garlic powder, paprika, and Italian seasoning). Simmer until the chicken is cooked through and the quinoa is tender, adding more broth if necessary. Serve hot with a sprinkle of fresh herbs, such as parsley or basil, for added flavor.

- Shrimp and Orzo Skillet: Sauté shrimp, diced tomatoes, spinach, garlic, and cooked orzo pasta in a skillet with olive oil until the shrimp are pink and opaque. Season with salt, pepper, and crushed red pepper flakes for a touch of heat. Garnish with grated Parmesan cheese and fresh lemon zest before serving for a burst of flavor.

- Beef and Mushroom Risotto: Brown ground beef or diced steak in a large pot or Dutch oven, then add sliced mushrooms, diced onion, minced garlic, Arborio rice, beef broth, and a splash of red wine. Simmer until the rice is creamy and tender, stirring occasionally. Stir in grated Parmesan cheese and chopped parsley before serving for a comforting and satisfying dinner.

These one-pot meals are not only quick to prepare but also offer a complete and balanced meal in a single dish, making cleanup a breeze.

Quick Stir-Fries and Skillet Dinners

Stir-fries and skillet dinners are versatile and flavorful options that come together quickly on busy evenings. Here are three quick stir-fry and skillet dinner ideas for seniors:

- Vegetable Stir-Fry with Tofu: Sauté diced tofu, bell peppers, snap peas, carrots, broccoli florets, and sliced mushrooms in a large skillet with sesame oil and soy sauce until the vegetables are tender-crisp and the tofu is lightly browned. Serve over cooked brown rice or quinoa for a nutritious and satisfying meal.

- Lemon Garlic Chicken Skillet: Sauté chicken breast cutlets in a skillet with olive oil, minced garlic, lemon zest, and lemon juice until golden brown and cooked through. Remove the chicken from the skillet and set aside. In the same skillet, add sliced cherry tomatoes and baby spinach, and cook until wilted. Return the chicken to the skillet and heat through. Serve hot with a side of steamed green beans or roasted potatoes for a flavorful dinner option.

- Beef and Broccoli Stir-Fry: Stir-fry thinly sliced beef sirloin with broccoli florets, sliced bell peppers, diced onion, and minced garlic in a wok or large skillet with sesame oil and oyster sauce until the beef is cooked to your desired doneness and the vegetables are tender-crisp. Serve over cooked rice or noodles for a hearty and satisfying meal.

These quick stir-fry and skillet dinner ideas are perfect for busy evenings when you need a nutritious and flavorful meal in a hurry.

Instant Pot and Slow Cooker Recipes for Easy Dinners

Instant Pot and slow cooker recipes offer hands-off cooking solutions that yield tender and flavorful dinners with minimal effort. Here are three Instant Pot and slow cooker recipes for easy dinners:

- Instant Pot Chicken and Vegetable Soup: Combine diced chicken breast, mixed vegetables, diced potatoes, onion, garlic, chicken broth, and herbs (such as thyme, rosemary, and bay leaves) in the Instant Pot. Cook on high pressure for 10 minutes, then allow the pressure to release naturally for 10 minutes before opening the lid. Serve hot with a slice of crusty whole grain bread for a comforting and nutritious dinner.

- Slow Cooker Beef Chili: Brown ground beef or turkey in a skillet, then transfer to a slow cooker along with diced tomatoes, kidney beans, black beans, diced onion, bell pepper, minced garlic, chili powder, cumin, and paprika. Cook on low for 6-8 hours or high for 3-4 hours, until flavors meld and chili thickens. Serve hot with a dollop of Greek yogurt or shredded cheese for added creaminess.

- Instant Pot Lentil Curry: Sauté diced onion, garlic, ginger, and curry paste in the Instant Pot with olive oil until fragrant. Add dried lentils, diced tomatoes, coconut milk, vegetable broth, and diced sweet potatoes. Cook on high pressure for 10 minutes, then quick release the pressure. Stir in chopped spinach and lime juice before serving for a flavorful and comforting curry.

These Instant Pot and slow cooker recipes offer convenient and hands-off cooking solutions that result in delicious and nutritious dinners with minimal effort required.

Incorporate these fast and flavorful dinner ideas into your evening routine to enjoy delicious and nutritious meals that support your diabetes management goals. With a variety of options to choose from, you can savor satisfying dinners without spending hours in the kitchen.

CHAPTER SIX

Snacks in Seconds for Between Meals

When managing diabetes, it's crucial to have quick and convenient snack options on hand to prevent blood sugar fluctuations between meals. These snacks should be nutrient-dense, satisfying, and easy to prepare. This section explores three categories of snacks in seconds for between meals: nutrient-dense snacks to tame hunger quickly, homemade snacks for healthy grazing, and portable snacks for on-the-go convenience.

Nutrient-Dense Snacks to Tame Hunger Quickly

Nutrient-dense snacks provide a quick energy boost while helping to stabilize blood sugar levels. Here are three options that can be prepared in seconds:

- Greek Yogurt with Berries: Top a serving of Greek yogurt with fresh or frozen berries for a satisfying snack that's rich in protein, calcium, and antioxidants. Greek yogurt contains probiotics that support gut health, while berries provide fiber and essential vitamins.

- Cottage Cheese and Fruit: Enjoy a serving of cottage cheese paired with sliced fruit, such as apples, pears, or peaches. Cottage cheese is high in protein and low in carbohydrates, making it an excellent option for managing blood sugar levels. The addition of fruit adds natural sweetness and additional nutrients.

- Almonds or Mixed Nuts: Grab a handful of almonds or mixed nuts for a quick and convenient snack that's rich in healthy fats, protein, and fiber. Nuts provide sustained energy and help keep hunger at bay between meals. Opt for unsalted varieties to control sodium intake.

These nutrient-dense snacks are simple to prepare and perfect for taming hunger quickly without causing blood sugar spikes.

Homemade Snacks for Healthy Grazing

Homemade snacks offer the advantage of being customizable and free from added sugars and preservatives. Here are three homemade snack ideas that can be prepared in seconds:

- Veggie Sticks with Hummus: Slice raw vegetables such as carrots, cucumbers, bell peppers, and celery into sticks and serve with a side of hummus for dipping. Hummus is made from chickpeas, which are rich in protein and fiber, while vegetables provide essential vitamins and minerals.

- Whole Grain Crackers with Cheese: Top whole grain crackers with slices of cheese for a satisfying and portable snack. Cheese is a good source of protein and calcium, while whole grain crackers provide fiber and complex carbohydrates.

Choose low-fat cheese options to keep saturated fat intake in check.

- Homemade Trail Mix: Mix together a variety of nuts, seeds, and dried fruits to create your own customized trail mix. Combine almonds, walnuts, pumpkin seeds, sunflower seeds, and dried cranberries or raisins for a balanced snack that provides protein, healthy fats, and carbohydrates.

These homemade snacks are quick to assemble and offer a nutritious alternative to store-bought options.

Portable Snacks for On-the-Go Convenience

Portable snacks are essential for busy days when you need a quick pick-me-up while on the move. Here are three portable snack options that can be enjoyed anywhere:

- Hard-Boiled Eggs: Prepare a batch of hard-boiled eggs in advance and store them in the refrigerator for a convenient grab-and-go snack. Eggs are rich in protein and essential nutrients, making them an excellent choice for managing blood sugar levels.

- Apple Slices with Peanut Butter: Slice an apple and serve with a single-serve packet of peanut butter for a satisfying and portable snack. Apples are high in fiber and antioxidants, while peanut butter provides protein and healthy fats.

Choose natural peanut butter without added sugars or hydrogenated oils.

- Greek Yogurt Parfait: Layer Greek yogurt with granola and sliced fruit in a portable container for a nutritious and delicious snack on the go. Greek yogurt provides protein and probiotics, while granola adds crunch and whole grains. Customize your parfait with your favorite fruits and toppings.

These portable snacks are convenient for carrying in a purse or backpack and offer a convenient way to curb hunger while away from home.

Incorporate these snacks in seconds into your daily routine to maintain energy levels and stabilize blood sugar throughout the day. With a variety of options to choose from, you can enjoy quick and convenient snacks that support your diabetes management goals.

CHAPTER SEVEN

Speedy Desserts for Sweet Cravings

When sweet cravings strike, it's important to have quick and satisfying dessert options that won't derail your efforts to manage diabetes. Speedy desserts should be lower in sugar, incorporate natural sweetness, and be easy to prepare. This section explores three categories of speedy desserts for sweet cravings: lower-sugar dessert recipes for seniors, fruit-based desserts for natural sweetness, and microwave mug cakes and no-bake treats.

Lower-Sugar Dessert Recipes for Seniors

Lower-sugar dessert recipes are ideal for seniors managing diabetes, providing a sweet treat without causing significant spikes in blood sugar levels. Here are three options that are quick to prepare:

- Greek Yogurt Parfait: Layer Greek yogurt with sliced strawberries or raspberries and a sprinkle of granola or crushed nuts for added texture. Greek yogurt is high in protein and lower in sugar than flavored yogurts, making it a healthier option for dessert. Customize your parfait with your favorite fruits and toppings.

- Dark Chocolate-Dipped Fruit: Melt dark chocolate chips in the microwave or over a double boiler, then dip sliced fruit such as bananas, strawberries, or oranges into the melted chocolate. Place the chocolate-dipped fruit on a parchment-lined baking sheet and refrigerate until the chocolate sets. Dark chocolate contains less sugar than milk chocolate and is rich in antioxidants, making it a healthier choice for dessert.

- Baked Apples with Cinnamon: Core and slice apples, then sprinkle with cinnamon and a drizzle of honey or maple syrup. Bake in the oven until the apples are tender and caramelized. Serve warm with a dollop of Greek yogurt or a scoop of low-sugar vanilla ice cream for a comforting and satisfying dessert.

These lower-sugar dessert recipes offer a sweet treat without causing significant fluctuations in blood sugar levels, making them suitable for seniors managing diabetes.

Fruit-Based Desserts for Natural Sweetness

Fruit-based desserts harness the natural sweetness of fruit to satisfy sweet cravings without the need for added sugars. Here are three options that are quick and easy to prepare:

- Mixed Berry Salad: Toss together a variety of fresh berries, such as strawberries, blueberries, raspberries, and blackberries, in a bowl. Drizzle with a squeeze of lemon juice and a sprinkle of fresh mint leaves for added flavor. Serve chilled for a refreshing and naturally sweet dessert option.

- Grilled Pineapple with Coconut Yogurt: Slice fresh pineapple into rings and grill until caramelized and slightly charred. Serve the grilled pineapple with a dollop of coconut yogurt and a sprinkle of toasted coconut flakes for a tropical-inspired dessert that's bursting with flavor.

- Frozen Banana Bites: Slice ripe bananas into coins and spread them out on a parchment-lined baking sheet. Dip each banana slice into melted dark chocolate, then sprinkle with chopped nuts or shredded coconut. Freeze until the chocolate sets, then serve cold for a refreshing and satisfying dessert.

These fruit-based desserts are not only quick and easy to prepare but also provide essential vitamins, minerals, and antioxidants, making them a healthy choice for satisfying sweet cravings.

Microwave Mug Cakes and No-Bake Treats

Microwave mug cakes and no-bake treats offer instant gratification without the need for lengthy baking or chilling times. Here are three options that are ready in minutes:

- Microwave Chocolate Mug Cake: Mix together flour, cocoa powder, baking powder, a pinch of salt, and a sweetener such as stevia or erythritol in a microwave-safe mug. Add milk, oil, and vanilla extract, then stir until smooth. Microwave on high for 1-2 minutes, or until the cake is set.

Serve warm with a dollop of Greek yogurt or whipped cream for a decadent dessert.

- No-Bake Energy Bites: Combine rolled oats, peanut butter, honey or maple syrup, and mix-ins such as chocolate chips, dried fruit, or chopped nuts in a bowl. Roll the mixture into bite-sized balls and refrigerate until firm. These energy bites are perfect for satisfying sweet cravings while providing a boost of energy and nutrition.

- Microwave Rice Krispie Treats: Melt butter in a microwave-safe bowl, then stir in marshmallows until melted and smooth. Add Rice Krispies cereal and stir until well coated. Press the mixture into a greased baking dish or divide it among individual muffin cups. Microwave on high for 1-2 minutes, or until set. Allow to cool before slicing into squares or removing from muffin cups.

These microwave mug cakes and no-bake treats offer quick and convenient dessert options that are perfect for satisfying sweet cravings in seconds.

Incorporate these speedy dessert ideas into your meal plan to enjoy sweet treats without compromising your efforts to manage diabetes. With a variety of options to choose from, you can indulge in delicious desserts that satisfy your cravings while supporting your health goals.

CHAPTER EIGHT

Side Dishes in a Flash

Side dishes play a crucial role in rounding out a meal, adding flavor, texture, and nutrients to the plate. For seniors managing diabetes, quick and convenient side dishes are essential for maintaining a balanced diet. This section explores three categories of side dishes in a flash: quick and delicious vegetable side dishes, simple whole grain and legume sides, and creative ways to prepare side dishes quickly.

Quick and Delicious Vegetable Side Dishes

Vegetables are a cornerstone of a healthy diet, providing essential vitamins, minerals, and fiber. Here are three quick and delicious vegetable side dishes that can be prepared in minutes:

- Sautéed Garlic Green Beans: Heat olive oil in a skillet over medium heat, then add trimmed green beans and minced garlic. Sauté until the green beans are tender-crisp and the garlic is fragrant, about 5-7 minutes. Season with salt, pepper, and a squeeze of lemon juice before serving for a flavorful and nutritious side dish.

- Roasted Brussels Sprouts with Balsamic Glaze: Toss halved Brussels sprouts with olive oil, salt, and pepper, then spread them out on a baking sheet. Roast in a preheated oven at 400°F (200°C) for 20-25 minutes, or until caramelized and tender. Drizzle with balsamic glaze before serving for a sweet and tangy twist on a classic side dish.

- Steamed Broccoli with Parmesan Cheese: Steam broccoli florets until tender, then toss with grated Parmesan cheese, lemon zest, and a sprinkle of red pepper flakes for added heat. Serve hot for a simple yet flavorful vegetable side dish that pairs well with any main course.

These quick and delicious vegetable side dishes are perfect for adding color and nutrition to your meals without spending hours in the kitchen.

Simple Whole Grain and Legume Sides

Whole grains and legumes are nutritious staples that provide complex carbohydrates, protein, and fiber. Here are three simple side dishes featuring whole grains and legumes that can be prepared in minutes:

- Quinoa Pilaf: Cook quinoa according to package instructions, then fluff with a fork and stir in diced vegetables such as bell peppers, onions, and carrots. Season with herbs and spices such as parsley, thyme, and garlic powder for added flavor. Serve hot as a nutrient-rich side dish or base for protein.

- Black Bean Salad: Rinse and drain canned black beans, then toss with diced tomatoes, red onion, bell peppers, cilantro, lime juice, and a drizzle of olive oil. Season with salt, pepper, and cumin for a refreshing and colorful side dish that's packed with protein and fiber.

- Brown Rice with Toasted Almonds: Cook brown rice according to package instructions, then fluff with a fork and stir in toasted slivered almonds and chopped fresh herbs such as parsley or chives. Season with salt and pepper to taste and serve hot as a wholesome and satisfying side dish.

These simple whole grain and legume sides are quick to prepare and offer a nutritious complement to any meal.

Creative Ways to Prepare Side Dishes Quickly

Get creative in the kitchen with these innovative ideas for preparing side dishes quickly:

- Veggie Noodle Stir-Fry: Use a spiralizer or vegetable peeler to create noodles from zucchini, carrots, or sweet potatoes. Stir-fry the veggie noodles with your favorite sauce and protein for a quick and healthy alternative to traditional pasta dishes.

- Sheet Pan Roasted Vegetables: Toss chopped vegetables such as bell peppers, onions, mushrooms, and cherry tomatoes with olive oil, salt, and pepper, then spread them out on a baking sheet. Roast in a preheated oven at 425°F (220°C) for 20-25 minutes, or until caramelized and tender, for a hands-off side dish that requires minimal effort.

- Instant Pot Beans and Rice: Combine rinsed and drained canned beans, uncooked rice, diced tomatoes, broth, and seasonings in an Instant Pot. Cook on high pressure for the recommended time, then allow the pressure to release naturally. Fluff with a fork and serve hot as a quick and hearty side dish.

These creative ways to prepare side dishes quickly offer versatility and convenience, allowing you to enjoy a variety of flavors and textures with minimal time and effort.

Incorporate these side dishes in a flash into your meal planning to add variety and nutrition to your meals without sacrificing time or convenience. With a little creativity and planning, you can enjoy delicious and nutritious side dishes that complement your main course and support your diabetes management goals.

CHAPTER NINE

Breakfast for Dinner: Brinner Ideas

Sometimes, a breakfast for dinner, or "brinner," can be just the comforting and satisfying meal you need, especially for seniors managing diabetes who may benefit from lighter evening meals. Brinner combines the best of both worlds – the flavors of breakfast with the heartiness of dinner. This section explores three categories of brinner ideas: savory breakfast dishes transformed into dinners, easy and quick breakfast casseroles, and breakfast burritos and frittatas for dinner.

Savory Breakfast Dishes Transformed into Dinners

Savory breakfast dishes can easily be transformed into hearty dinners by adding a few extra ingredients or swapping out traditional breakfast components. Here are three ideas to get you started:

- Breakfast Hash: Start with diced potatoes sautéed until golden brown, then add diced bell peppers, onions, and any leftover cooked vegetables you have on hand. Mix in cooked breakfast sausage or crumbled bacon for protein, and finish with a sprinkle of shredded cheese and a fried or poached egg on top. Serve hot with a side of whole grain toast for a satisfying brinner option.

- Quiche with Mixed Greens Salad: Bake a quiche using a pre-made crust or crustless option filled with a mixture of eggs, milk, cheese, and your choice of vegetables and protein, such as spinach, mushrooms, ham, or smoked salmon. Serve slices of quiche with a mixed greens salad dressed with vinaigrette for a balanced and flavorful dinner.

- Breakfast Pizza: Start with a pre-made pizza crust or flatbread, then spread with marinara sauce and sprinkle with shredded cheese. Top with cooked breakfast ingredients such as scrambled eggs, crumbled sausage, diced bell peppers, and sliced mushrooms. Bake until the cheese is melted and bubbly, then garnish with chopped fresh herbs like parsley or chives before serving.

These savory breakfast dishes transformed into dinners offer a delicious and comforting option for a brinner meal.

Easy and Quick Breakfast Casseroles

Breakfast casseroles are a convenient way to enjoy a hearty meal that can be prepared in advance and reheated for dinner. Here are three easy and quick breakfast casserole ideas for brinner:

- Spinach and Feta Egg Bake: Whisk together eggs, milk, crumbled feta cheese, chopped spinach, diced onion, and minced garlic in a baking dish. Bake until set and golden brown, then slice into squares and serve hot with a side of whole grain bread or a mixed greens salad for a satisfying brinner option.

- Sausage and Hash Brown Casserole: Layer cooked breakfast sausage, frozen hash browns, diced bell peppers, onions, and shredded cheese in a baking dish. Whisk together eggs, milk, and seasonings such as salt, pepper, and paprika, then pour over the sausage and hash brown mixture. Bake until the eggs are set and the top is golden brown, then slice and serve hot for a hearty brinner option.

- French Toast Casserole: Arrange slices of day-old bread in a baking dish, then pour a mixture of eggs, milk, vanilla extract, and cinnamon over the bread, ensuring that each slice is coated. Sprinkle with a mixture of brown sugar and chopped nuts, then bake until golden brown and crispy. Serve hot with a drizzle of maple syrup or a dollop of Greek yogurt for a sweet and satisfying brinner option.

These easy and quick breakfast casseroles are perfect for brinner and can be customized with your favorite ingredients for endless variations.

Breakfast Burritos and Frittatas for Dinner

Breakfast burritos and frittatas are versatile options that can be enjoyed for dinner with a variety of fillings and toppings. Here are three ideas to try:

- Breakfast Burritos: Fill whole grain tortillas with scrambled eggs, cooked breakfast sausage or bacon, diced potatoes, shredded cheese, and salsa. Roll up the burritos tightly, then grill or pan-fry until crispy and golden brown. Serve hot with a side of avocado slices or Greek yogurt for dipping.

- Veggie Frittata: Sauté diced vegetables such as bell peppers, onions, mushrooms, and spinach in an oven-safe skillet until tender. Whisk together eggs, milk, shredded cheese, and seasonings, then pour over the vegetables in the skillet. Cook on the stovetop until the edges are set, then transfer to the oven and bake until the frittata is golden brown and puffed up. Serve hot with a side of mixed greens salad for a nutritious brinner option.

- Smoked Salmon and Asparagus Frittata: Arrange blanched asparagus spears and smoked salmon slices in an oven-safe skillet, then pour whisked eggs, milk, and chopped fresh dill over the top. Sprinkle with shredded cheese and season with salt and pepper. Cook on the stovetop until the edges are set, then transfer to the oven and bake until the frittata is cooked through. Serve hot with a squeeze of lemon juice for a flavorful and elegant brinner option.

These breakfast burritos and frittatas for dinner offer a delicious and satisfying option for brinner that can be customized to suit your taste preferences.

Incorporate these brinner ideas into your meal planning to enjoy a comforting and satisfying meal that combines the best of breakfast and dinner. With a variety of options to choose from, you can indulge in delicious brinner meals that support your diabetes management goals.

CHAPTER TEN

Meal Prep Tips for Quick and Healthy Eating

Meal prep is a game-changer when it comes to maintaining a healthy diet, especially for seniors managing diabetes. By dedicating some time to preparation in advance, you can ensure that nutritious meals are always within reach, even on busy days. This section explores three categories of meal prep tips for quick and healthy eating: time-saving meal prep strategies after 50, batch cooking and freezing meals for convenience, and tips for efficient grocery shopping and ingredient prep.

Time-Saving Meal Prep Strategies After 50

As we age, time-saving strategies become increasingly important to help manage busy schedules while maintaining a healthy diet. Here are three time-saving meal prep strategies for seniors after 50:

- Plan Your Meals: Take some time at the beginning of each week to plan out your meals and snacks. Consider your schedule, dietary preferences, and nutritional needs when choosing recipes. Make a shopping list based on your meal plan to ensure you have all the ingredients on hand.

- Prep Ingredients in Advance: Spend some time prepping ingredients in advance to streamline the cooking process. Wash, chop, and portion out vegetables, fruits, and proteins such as chicken or tofu. Store prepped ingredients in airtight containers or resealable bags in the refrigerator for easy access throughout the week.

- Use Time-Saving Kitchen Tools: Invest in kitchen tools and gadgets that can help you save time during meal prep. Consider using a slow cooker, Instant Pot, or food processor to simplify cooking tasks such as chopping, sautéing, and simmering. Opt for pre-cut or pre-washed produce to cut down on prep time even further.

These time-saving meal prep strategies can help seniors after 50 enjoy nutritious meals without spending hours in the kitchen each day.

Batch Cooking and Freezing Meals for Convenience

Batch cooking and freezing meals in advance is a convenient way to ensure that you always have healthy options on hand, especially on busy days. Here are three tips for batch cooking and freezing meals for convenience:

- Choose Freezer-Friendly Recipes: Look for recipes that freeze well and can be reheated easily, such as soups, stews, casseroles, and pasta dishes. Prepare large batches of these recipes and portion them out into individual servings before freezing. Label each container with the name of the dish and the date it was prepared for easy identification.

- Use Freezer Bags for Portioning: Consider using freezer bags instead of containers for portioning out meals. Freezer bags are space-saving and allow you to lay meals flat for efficient storage. Be sure to remove as much air as possible from the bags before sealing to prevent freezer burn.

- Reheat Safely: When reheating frozen meals, ensure that they reach an internal temperature of 165°F (74°C) to kill any bacteria and ensure food safety. Use a microwave, oven, or stovetop to reheat frozen meals, following the recommended cooking instructions for each dish.

By batch cooking and freezing meals in advance, seniors can enjoy the convenience of having nutritious meals ready to go whenever they need them.

Tips for Efficient Grocery Shopping and Ingredient Prep

Efficient grocery shopping and ingredient prep are key components of successful meal prep. Here are three tips for seniors to streamline the grocery shopping and ingredient prep process:

- Make a Shopping List: Before heading to the grocery store, make a list of the ingredients you'll need for your planned meals and snacks. Organize your list by category (e.g., produce, dairy, pantry staples) to make shopping more efficient. Consider using grocery shopping apps or online ordering for added convenience.

- Shop the Perimeter: When navigating the grocery store, focus on shopping the perimeter where fresh produce, meats, dairy, and whole grains are typically located. Limit the amount of time spent in the center aisles, which tend to contain processed and packaged foods that may be less nutritious.

- Prep Ingredients Right Away: After returning from the grocery store, take some time to prep ingredients right away before storing them in the refrigerator or pantry. Wash and chop fruits and vegetables, portion out snacks into individual servings, and prepare any marinades or sauces in advance. This will make meal prep throughout the week much quicker and easier.

By implementing these tips for efficient grocery shopping and ingredient prep, seniors can save time and ensure they have everything they need to create healthy and delicious meals at home.

Incorporate these meal prep tips into your routine to enjoy quick and healthy eating with minimal effort. With a little planning and preparation, you can maintain a nutritious diet that supports your diabetes management goals while still enjoying delicious meals and snacks.

CHAPTER 12

31 DAY MEAL PLAN

Week 1:

Day 1:

- Breakfast: Whole grain toast with avocado slices and a poached egg.

- Lunch: Spinach and chicken salad with cherry tomatoes and balsamic vinaigrette.

- Dinner: Grilled salmon with steamed broccoli.

Day 2:

- Breakfast: Greek yogurt with mixed berries and a sprinkle of cinnamon.

- Lunch: Turkey and cheese roll-up with lettuce and mustard.

- Dinner: Stir-fried tofu with mixed vegetables.

Day 3:

- Breakfast: Oatmeal topped with sliced bananas and a drizzle of honey.

- Lunch: Tuna salad with cucumber and carrot sticks.

- Dinner: Baked chicken breast with roasted Brussels sprouts.

Day 4:

- Breakfast: Smoothie with spinach, almond milk, banana, and protein powder.

- Lunch: Quinoa salad with diced bell peppers, cucumber, and feta cheese.

- Dinner: Shrimp stir-fry with snap peas and brown rice.

Day 5:

- Breakfast: Cottage cheese with peach slices and a sprinkle of chopped nuts.

- Lunch: Black bean and corn salad with avocado and lime dressing.

- Dinner: Grilled steak with a side of grilled asparagus.

Week 2:

Day 6:

- Breakfast: Whole grain waffles with Greek yogurt and sliced strawberries.

- Lunch: Chicken Caesar salad with homemade dressing.

- Dinner: Baked cod with lemon and herbs, served with sautéed spinach.

Day 7:

- Breakfast: Scrambled eggs with diced bell peppers and onions.

- Lunch: Veggie wrap with hummus, lettuce, and tomato.

- Dinner: Turkey meatballs in marinara sauce with spaghetti squash.

Day 8:

- Breakfast: Whole grain toast with almond butter and apple slices.

- Lunch: Lentil soup with a side of mixed greens.

- Dinner: Grilled pork chops with roasted carrots.

Day 9:

- Breakfast: Smoothie bowl with mixed berries, almond milk, and granola.

- Lunch: Caprese salad with sliced tomatoes, mozzarella, and basil.

- Dinner: Baked tilapia with steamed green beans.

Day 10:

- Breakfast: Yogurt parfait with granola and sliced peaches.

- Lunch: Turkey and avocado wrap with lettuce and tomato.

- Dinner: Stir-fried beef with broccoli and brown rice.

Week 3:

Day 11:

- Breakfast: Whole grain cereal with low-fat milk and sliced bananas.

- Lunch: Spinach and feta stuffed chicken breast.

- Dinner: Grilled salmon with roasted asparagus.

Day 12:

- Breakfast: Egg muffins with spinach, mushrooms, and cheese.

- Lunch: Chickpea salad with cucumber, tomatoes, and olives.

- Dinner: Baked chicken thighs with roasted cauliflower.

Day 13:

- Breakfast: Overnight oats with almond milk, chia seeds, and berries.

- Lunch: Turkey lettuce wraps with sliced bell peppers.

- Dinner: Shrimp and vegetable stir-fry with quinoa.

Day 14:

- Breakfast: Whole grain pancakes with Greek yogurt and mixed berries.
- Lunch: Caesar salad with grilled chicken breast.
- Dinner: Baked cod with roasted Brussels sprouts.

Day 15:

- Breakfast: Cottage cheese with pineapple chunks and a sprinkle of cinnamon.
- Lunch: Greek salad with feta cheese, olives, and cucumbers.
- Dinner: Grilled steak with sautéed spinach.

Week 4:

Day 16:

- Breakfast: Smoothie with spinach, mango, almond milk, and protein powder.
- Lunch: Turkey and cheese roll-up with lettuce and mustard.
- Dinner: Stir-fried tofu with broccoli and brown rice.

Day 17:

- Breakfast: Whole grain toast with avocado slices and a poached egg.

- Lunch: Tuna salad with cucumber and carrot sticks.

- Dinner: Grilled chicken breast with steamed broccoli.

Day 18:

- Breakfast: Omelette with diced bell peppers, onions, and cheese.

- Lunch: Spinach and strawberry salad with balsamic vinaigrette.

- Dinner: Baked salmon with roasted asparagus.

Day 19:

- Breakfast: Greek yogurt with mixed berries and a drizzle of honey.

- Lunch: Black bean and corn salad with avocado and lime dressing.

- Dinner: Grilled pork chops with roasted carrots.

Day 20:

- Breakfast: Whole grain waffles with Greek yogurt and sliced strawberries.

- Lunch: Caprese salad with sliced tomatoes, mozzarella, and basil.

- Dinner: Turkey meatballs in marinara sauce with spaghetti squash.

Week 5:

Day 21:

- Breakfast: Whole grain cereal with low-fat milk and sliced bananas.

- Lunch: Veggie wrap with hummus, lettuce, and tomato.

- Dinner: Baked tilapia with steamed green beans.

Day 22:

- Breakfast: Yogurt parfait with granola and sliced peaches.

- Lunch: Caesar salad with grilled chicken breast.

- Dinner: Stir-fried beef with broccoli and brown rice.

Day 23:

- Breakfast: Whole grain pancakes with Greek yogurt and mixed berries.

- Lunch: Turkey lettuce wraps with sliced bell peppers.

- Dinner: Shrimp and vegetable stir-fry with quinoa.

Day 24:

- Breakfast: Egg muffins with spinach, mushrooms, and cheese.

- Lunch: Chickpea salad with cucumber, tomatoes, and olives.

- Dinner: Baked chicken thighs with roasted cauliflower.

Day 25:

- Breakfast: Overnight oats with almond milk, chia seeds, and berries.

- Lunch: Spinach and feta stuffed chicken breast.

- Dinner: Grilled salmon with roasted asparagus.

Week 6:

Day 26:

- Breakfast: Smoothie with spinach, mango, almond milk, and protein powder.

- Lunch: Turkey and cheese roll-up with lettuce and mustard.

- Dinner: Stir-fried tofu with broccoli and brown rice.

Day 27:

- Breakfast: Whole grain toast with avocado slices and a poached egg.

- Lunch: Tuna salad with cucumber and carrot sticks.

- Dinner: Grilled chicken breast with steamed broccoli.

Day 28:

- Breakfast: Omelette with diced bell peppers, onions, and cheese.

- Lunch: Spinach and strawberry salad with balsamic vinaigrette.

- Dinner: Baked salmon with roasted asparagus.

Day 29:

- Breakfast: Greek yogurt with mixed berries and a drizzle of honey.

- Lunch: Black bean and corn salad with avocado and lime dressing.

- Dinner: Grilled pork chops with roasted carrots.

Day 30:

- Breakfast: Whole grain waffles with Greek yogurt and sliced strawberries.

- Lunch: Caprese salad with sliced tomatoes, mozzarella, and basil.

- Dinner: Turkey meatballs in marinara sauce with spaghetti squash.

Day 31:

- Breakfast: Whole grain cereal with low-fat milk and sliced bananas.

- Lunch: Veggie wrap with hummus, lettuce, and tomato.

- Dinner: Baked tilapia with steamed green beans.

THE END